Self-Mutilation, Suicide, and Homicide:
It is in Your DNA
Your 9th Psychiatric Consultation.
William R. Yee M.D., J.D.
Copyright Applied for 02/29/2020

Childhood is Confusing:because of the lack of context.

Thus, the many, "why's," of childhood.

Alexander the Great, was born July 20, 356 B.C. died June 10, 323 BC and caused 3.5 million people to die.

Genghis Khan, (1162, died August 18, 1227), caused the death of 40 million people or 10% of the world's population.

Adolf Hitler, born April 20, 1889, died April 30, 1945 caused the death 75 million people in World War II.

Chairman Mao, Mao Zedong, born December 26, 1893, died September 9, 1976, was responsible for as many as 110 million deaths.

It is now known that there is a relationship between suicide and homicide.

That is why there are so many stories of a combination of suicide and homicide in the news, captioned as, "murder-suicide," in the lay press.

Context develops further as follows:
Kelly Girl Service, Inc. was established in in 1946 and is headquartered in Troy, Michigan.

First Encounters
1949

In 1949, António Egas Moniz received the Nobel Prize in medicine for his development of the prefrontal lobotomy.

Violent, assaultive, and self-mutilating behavior now had a surgical procedure for treatment.

At that time treatment of mental illness, self-mutilation, suicide, and homicidal behaviors included wrapping patients in wet sheets and putting them in baths of ice water, insulin shock therapy, and electroconvulsive therapy.

Insulin shock therapy was hard to control and dangerous.

It is difficult to control the blood sugar levels with high doses of insulin.

If the blood level falls below 40 there can be permanent damage in addition to the seizures.

Permanent damage includes death, or death of the cerebral hemispheres.

With death of the cerebral hemispheres, all that is left is the brainstem.

The heart beats, and the patient breaths, because the brain stem survives.
The patient never wakes up, and never talks again.

The patient remains in this vegetative state, with a heart that beats, and lungs that breath, but in a permanent coma until death.

Lobotomy was believed to be the only effective treatment for severe mental illness manifesting self-mutilation, assault, homicide, and suicidal behaviors.

To perform a lobotomy the "surgeon," pushes an ice pick into the eye socket next to the eyeball.

The lacrimal ducts were often used as the starting point.

The surgeon continues pushing the icepick through the bone into the brain.

He then waves the pick back and forth to sever connections between the frontal lobe of the brain and other parts of the brain.

The effect of the prefrontal lobotomy was inconsistent as it was a crude procedure by any standard.

For more information and a report by one of the many who had a lobotomy see:

He was bad, so they put an ice pick in his brain..., Elizabeth Day, The Guardian, The Obser1633-1637 ver Neuroscience, Sun 13 Jan 2008 18.40 EST, https://www.theguardian.com/science/2008/jan/13/neuroscience.medicalscience

Howard Dully describes his memory of having a lobotomy at the age of 12.

He describes his life before and after the lobotomy.

This article has an excellent review of how Dr Walter Freeman brought the lobotomy to America in the late 1930s for the treatment of mental illness.

The rise and demise of the lobotomy due to use and abuse is also discussed.

The use and abuse of psychiatric treatments is a common pattern among psychiatric treatments, as their limited use in research and carefully controlled academic settings migrates to widespread use and the commercial pressures of profit and marketing are applied.

The best and most recent examples are well defined by litigation regarding the use and abuse of oxycontin and fentanyl. The lawsuits against opioids are proliferating.
See:
"First opioid lawsuit settlement raises questions with dozens more cases waiting," David L. Noll, Opionds Rescource Center, April 3, 2019,

1951
Almost 20,000 medical lobotomies were performed for the treatment of mental illness.

The rise and demise of the lobotomy for the treatment of mental illness mirrors the rise and demise of the tulip mania in Holland, 1633 to1637, or the subprime mortgage crises of 2007 to 2010.
The reason is they were all subject to the same market forces and the same mathematics of Chaos Theory.

It all starts with high speculative expectations and ends in acrimonious recriminations.
For acrimonious recriminations regarding lobotomies and other medical procedures see:
"10 Awful Realities Behind The Lobotomy Craze," GREGORY MYERS, HUMANS |

There is a large literature hostile to lobotomies on the internet.

There are many attorney websites seeking clients to sue regarding just about every psychiatric treatment and medication.

1954
In 1954 Thorazine replaced surgical lobotomies.

Thorazine was quickly labeled a, "chemical lobotomy," with the, "Thorazine Shuffle," adding insult to injury.

Violent, assaultive, and self-mutilating behavior now had a medication for treatment.

1955
My first encounter with self-mutilation was in about 1955.
In 1955 I was living in the Shady Lane Trailer Park on Capital Street, by Nine Mile and Ryan in Warren, Michigan.

This was a suburb of Detroit.

My best friends were Roger and Steven Smith.

Their grandparents lived in West Virginia and their parents came to Detroit looking for work in the factories.

They were Baptists. I was a Seventh Day Adventist.

My mother sent us to Baptist Churches when there were no nearby Seventh Day Adventist churches.

My mother didn't see many differences among religions, and she thought that religious instruction in the Golden Rule and the Ten Commandments was more important than any religious affiliation.

One day, Roger said, "we are best friends. We should be blood brothers."

"We should cut our thumbs and press them together."

"Our blood will mix, and we will be blood brothers."

I had seen this in western movies.

A cowboy and an Indian would become friends and then they would do this and become blood brothers.

I did not like the idea of cutting myself because I knew it would hurt.

I did not see anything wrong with cutting myself to be a blood brother with my best friends.

It made sense to me.
It was just like in the movies.

When Roger gave me the knife, I cut my thumb.

This was not simple.

The knife was sharp, but it was not as sharp as a razor.

The first few times it did not cut deep enough to draw blood, but it hurt each time.

If I cut to the bone, I would get a beating from my father.

I had to do it quickly, because Roger and Steven were there waiting, and I had to do it before their blood dried.

It took a few attempts, but I drew blood in less than a minute.

What a relief.

I pressed my thumb against Roger's thumb, then I pressed it against Steven's thumb.

My brother did the same and we were and are blood brothers.

Roger and Steven Smith remain family, although I have lost track of them and have not been able to find them.

Finding them is on my bucket list.

However, they were heavy smokers, and I may never be able to talk to them again.

A sad thought.

Since then I have had many other encounters with self-mutilation.

We had a neighbor across the road
between the rows of trailers.

It was a dirt road and too narrow to park
cars.

The neighbor would scratch his temples
from time to time as we talked.

He was self-conscious of this habit.

He had round pale pink spots on each side
of his face the size of a silver dollar.

They were the first thing you noticed
when you looked at his tanned, leathery
face.

He noticed that when we met, the first
thing I did was look at them.

I suppose most people did.
It was hard not to stare at the two large
round pink spots.

Although I was only eight years old, he
felt compelled to tell me,

"I have a nervous habit and I can't stop
scratching, no matter how hard I try."

He added,
"I have talked to doctors about it but there is nothing that they can do to help me stop scratching there."

1958
In 1958 I read <u>The Eternal Search; the Story of Man and his Drugs</u> by Richard R. Mathison.

This was the very first textbook in medicine that I ever read.

Mr. Mathison exposed me to centuries of bizarre behaviors used to treat medical illness.

What I found most strange was the use of feces for the treatment of medical illness.

People would actually eat feces as medicine.

People ate feces in many parts of the world for many centuries to cure various illnesses.

I suppose people are still eating feces in many places as medicine.

For my part, I don't think I could force myself to eat feces, but many people have done exactly that.

Feces as medicine, really?

The world is a truly a large and strange place for a child to explore.

I was not aware of the fact that in 1958 Ben Eiseman treated fulminant pseudomembranous colitis with fecal enemas with rapid return to health.

Mr. Mathison described other strange practices.

Bleeding by the knife and with leeches gave doctors the title of, "Leeches."

George Washington and many famous founders of this country were in fact bled by "leeches" when they were sick.

1960
Jeffrey Lionel Dahmer, born May 21, 1960.
1963
In high school around 1963, I met a very tall student who showed me scars on his forearm.

He told me how he got the scars.

"I bet someone that they could put a twenty- dollar bill on my forearm and burn a hole through it with a cigarette and I will not flinch."

"If I flinch and pull my arm away from the cigarette, I lose the bet. If I do not flinch, and let the cigarette burn a hole through the twenty-dollar bill to my skin I win the bet and keep the twenty-dollar bill. "

He was proud of the fact that,
"I have never lost a bet. I kept every twenty-dollar bill."

I knew that I would lose every bet like that.

I would draw my arm away before the hole was burnt through the twenty-dollar bill.

I felt very small and weak next to him.

I admired his ability to tolerate pain. I also knew that I was not going to try to improve my pain tolerance to that level.

I could control my scratching and not have a nervous habit that gave me large pink spots on my temples.

I could cut myself with a knife to be a blood brother with my friends.

I could not allow myself to be burned by a cigarette just to impress and win a bet.

When I was growing up there were war movies and I learned about Japanese kamikaze pilots who would kill themselves for family-honor.

I also learned that the Japanese would rather commit suicide than lose family-honor by surrendering.

I thought to myself that I could not commit suicide.

I thought that the Japanese had more courage than I did because they could commit suicide and I could not.

People are different and do things for different reasons.

I knew that since childhood.

I had a lot more to learn.

College 1965 to 1968

1965
In 1965 I started my first factory job for Chrysler at the Warren Stamping Plant 22800 Mound Rd, Warren, MI 48091. The plant opened in 1948 when I was one year old.

At that plant I met "Crusher," Cortez, the huge wrestler.

We both worked in the same section where the small portable stamping presses were placed.

I would punch out of the third shift. I would see him as he came in for the first shift at about 7:00 am.

Crusher Cortez was a professional wrestler for over thirty years, while working for Chrysler.

I never had the chance to talk to Crusher Cortez.
I often wondered why a famous professional wrestler would work in a factory during the week.

I met Roger Smith at the Warren Stamping plant.

He told me many things,
"I did an apprenticeship here. I am a journeyman tool and die maker. I make real good money."

"You should sign up for the apprenticeship. It would be easy for you and you would make a lot more money as a tool and die maker than running these presses."

"The work can be dangerous."

"People have been crushed to death by the dies."

"If you are careful, you won't get hurt."

I told Roger,

"I have a college scholarship and I am working for extra money to live on."

"I am not planning on working in a factory for twenty years and retiring with a pension."

Roger understood, but we talked from time to time, and he kept repeating the suggestion.

We were, "blood brothers," and he liked the thought of working with me until we both retired.

One of the sad things about making friends is that one rarely travels the same path with friends for a lifetime.

I have made many friends in many places, and have parted ways many times.

I hope my friends read this book and we may meet again, like in the TV program, "This is Your Life."

Roger was right about the job being dangerous.

People were having their fingers and hands cut off all the time.

The foreman and general foreman said. "they do it on purpose."

"They do it to get money to buy a Cadillac."

I wouldn't cut off a finger to buy a car. I didn't think that the other union members would either.

This was one of many dividing lines between union members and management.

I was eighteen and very fast on the job.

One day I was asked to leave my job to work on another machine.

There was my foreman, the union steward, the safety man, a general foreman and a union committee man, all there to watch me.

My foreman explained the situation to me, because the union rule was that only your foreman could give you orders and instructions

"A man just had his arm cut off by that machine because he reached through the die to pull the trim off."

"I want you to run the machine, but if the trim sticks to the die, you walk around behind the machine to pull the trim off."

"Don't reach through the die to pull the trim off."

I said,
"I will not reach through the die to pull the trim off. I don't want it to cut my arm off."

The machine was a small portable press.

It stamped out a part that was about three and a half, feet long, and an inch wide.

It had a T shaped stand in front of it with a red button on each side.

The design and set up of the press, the die and the red buttons that started the press for each cycle was designed for maximum ease and speed of production.

I was instructed to place a blank sheet of metal on the bottom part of the die.

Then I was to push the red buttons.

I was instructed to leave my hands on the red buttons and watch the top half of the die come down and rise back up.

When the top half of the die came done it struck the metal blank with enough force to shape it and cut off the excess metal when it hit the bottom half of the die.

When it rose up, it would stop.

Then I was instructed to take the stamping out of the die and put it into the basket of finished parts to be removed when full.

Then I was instructed to take the trim waste from the die and place it into the waste basket.

Sometimes the trim waste stuck to the die.

I could lean forward, over the T shaped stand with the red buttons, and over the die to pull the trim off.
When I reached over the die to pull off the trim two things happened.

The first thing was that I was off balance when I leaned forward. I could not quickly pull my arms back if the top die came done suddenly.

The second thing that happened was my elbows were above the red buttons, and could easily push them and start the cycle so that the top die would come down to cut my arms off while I was reaching through the die to pull the stuck waste trim off of the die.

I was working fast, and of course, the trim stuck to the die.

Without stopping to think, I reached through the die to pull the stuck trim off.

I was stopped.

"Don't reach through the die, walk around and pull the trim off from behind the machine."

I did as I was instructed.

I went back to work and after a while, the trim stuck to the die again.

Without thinking, I reached over the die to pull of the trim.
I was stopped and warned,
"If you reach over the die again you will be fired."

I answered,
"Yes, I understand. I don't want my arm
cut off either."

I went back to work and after a while
another piece of trim got stuck to the die
and without thinking I reached over the
die to pull it off."

Again, I was warned,
"I told you that if you reached over the
die you would be fired."

I answered,
"I know, but you get into a rhythm, and
you aren't thinking, it's like you are
hypnotized, and you reach over without
thinking."

I was not fired. The job was shut down,
and I was told to go back to my original
job assignment.

I did not see that trim-job operational for
about a month.
When it was started it had restraints so
your hands could not reach over the die.
It also had the red buttons placed above
the top die so your elbows could not push
them by accident and start the cycle.

It was reorganized for maximum safety and minimum production.

That is the Ying and Yang of reality.

Maximum one at the cost of the Minimum of the other.

The production rate dropped a lot with the new set up.

I don't think that man cut his arm off on purpose.

I don't think I reached over the die on purpose.

Working in a factory can be a dangerous job.

The division between management and union members is about money and safety.

Safety costs money and reduces profits. There are other possibilities.

1967
I saw the movie, <u>Bonnie and Clyde.</u>

Warren Beatty starred as Clyde, and Faye Dunaway starred as Bonnie.

In the opening scene Warren Beatty tells Faye Dunaway that he was limping because he cut off his toe.

He explains that he cut off his toe so he could go to the hospital.

He said that he thought that it would be easier to escape from a hospital than a prison.

Then he laughs and says he was let out of prison and did not have to escape.
Faye Dunaway tells Warren Beatty that she did not believe anything he was saying.

Warren Beatty is annoyed and robs a bank to impress Faye Dunaway and prove he is a criminal.
The point is that antisocial personalities will self-mutilate to create opportunity and to impress.

This is operational self-mutilation, and a product of prison culture, but not necessarily mental illness.

In college my favorite class was social anthropology.

Social anthropology is the study of variations in behavior between cultures.

Social anthropology explores the law, family, and economics in different cultures.

I saw extremes in marriage.

The range in family honor went from murder to suicide.

Eskimos would share their wives with guests.

Moslems would kill their wife and their wife's lover for family-honor.

A society in the Pacific would execute a murderer, and all of the murderer's relatives.
They did not build prisons.

In 1967 I started working at the the Chrysler Detroit Axle Plant (AKA the Eldon Axle Plant or the Eldon Avenue Gear and Axle Plant).

The Detroit Axle Plant (Eldon Avenue Gearand Axle Plant) was on 6700 Lynch Road in Detroit and Hamtramck.

The Eldon Avenue Gear and Axle plant opened in 1917, and closed in 2010, and has been demolished.

I was an inspector at the Eldon Gear and Axle plant from 1967 to 1971.

I really enjoyed my work at the Eldon Avenue gear and axle plant. I as an inspector. It was a lot easier than operating a press or being a tool and die maker.

I wasn't making as much money as a journeyman tool and die maker.

I was making over three dollars an hour and more money than I had ever made in my life.

I made over one hundred dollars after taxes for forty hours.
I made about one hundred and fifty dollars after taxes for forty-eight hours with Saturday paid at a rate of time and a half.

I made about one hundred and seventy-five dollars after taxes for fifty-six hours with double time on Sundays and time and a half on Saturdays.

I also enjoyed talking to all the people I met, except for the drug addict dealer who said to me,
"mind your own F*ing business, or I will kill your ass."

All I could say in response to that threat was,
"I didn't see anything."

For a different experience you should talk to Barry Stuart. If you can't talk to him, read what he said at;
http://carbon314.com/ghosts-of-eldon-avenue-2/

He paints a much different picture.

Barry didn't like working at the Chrysler Eldon Avenue Gear and Axle plant at all. You can be in the same place and live in a different world.

I realized that if you belong to a different culture, you can live in the same place and have a completely different experience.

That explained the difference between Union and Management in the auto factories.

That explained the difference between Barry's experience and my experience.

Barry was White Collar and I was Blue Collar by culture. We lived in different worlds.

During my stay there I met the peanut vendor, the porn vendor, the loan shark, the numbers runner, a variety of drug merchants, and I heard of pimps recruiting the young women.

I talked to them all, and I enjoyed the opportunity to look into many different worlds.
I saw employees who returned to work bruised and bandaged after they cashed their checks at nearby bars and were mugged.

I talked to the loan shark. He carried large wads of money.

On payday, Thursday, he would take checks and give people money.

I asked him,
"how much does it cost to borrow money from you?"

He said,
"it costs you15% a week to borrow money from me."

I asked him,
"what is the smallest amount of money that I can borrow?"

He said
"I will loan you five dollars."

"OK, loan me five dollars."

It would cost me seventy-five cents to borrow five dollars and have my check cashed the following week.

I was working and going to school, and it was hard to find time to go to a bank and cash my checks.

Every week I borrowed five dollars, and paid the loan shark seventy, five cents, to cash my check.

He knew what I was doing, but he didn't mind.

He was huge, six foot seven and two hundred and seventy pounds.

I was all of five foot five inches tall and one hundred and fifty pounds.

One day as I was cashing a check. I looked at his huge wad of bills.

I looked up, into his eyes, and said, "what if I decided to take that money from you?"

He smiled at me and said,

"I have friends with guns."

I said, "yeah, let's be friends."

I worked on the second shift in Department 72, where the rear axle housings were finished.

The second shift had a large contingent of gay and transgender males.

When they found out I was going to medical school, they asked me a lot of questions about gender change surgery.

I disappointed them. I said,
"I am going to medical school. I have a lot to learn. Ask again in maybe ten years."

Medical School 1968 to 1972
When I went to medical school, I learned about self-mutilation due to genetic defects.

Lesch–Nyhan disease is a disease caused by a genetic abnormality that results in self-mutilation.

The self-mutilation of Lesch–Nyhan disease is not a learned behavior.

The self-mutilation of Lesch–Nyhan disease is caused by a genetic abnormality that is inherited.

The patient with Lesch–Nyhan disease will pull out his eyeballs. He will chew off his lips and fingers.

He will spend his life with his hands restrained to his waist to keep them away from his eyes and his empty eye sockets to prevent continuing and persistent self-mutilation.

The patient with Lesch–Nyhan disease will have his teeth pulled so that he cannot continue to chew his lips and fingers off.

There is no effective treatment for the self-mutilation of Lesch–Nyhan disease. 1969

In 1969 I read the book On Death and Dying by Dr. Elisabeth Kübler-Ross.

She adds, "What the Dying Have to Teach Doctors, Nurses, Clergy and their Own Families," to her title and book cover.

Dr. Ross describes the stress of finding out about cancer as a grief that occurs in stages.

Denial – She has observed patients with cancer as first manifesting denial.

They cannot accept the death sentence.

My thoughts,
"The doctor made a mistake. The lab made a mistake. Another test, another doctor, a second opinion, anything...."

Anger –
Then she observes anger. My thoughts, "why me? I should have had better medical care. There should have been a cleaner work environment, anything...."

Bargaining –
She observes bargaining. My thoughts, ""If I give up alcohol and go to church can I live longer? please God? Anything..."

Depression –
She observes patients giving up and doing nothing. My thoughts,
"It's hopeless. There is nothing I can do. I will just give up. I won't do anything. I won't talk to anybody. I won't....

Acceptance –
Finally, she sees patients accepting cancer, accepting their death and making

the best of each of their remaining days.

My thoughts,
"OK, I don't have much time left and I
have a lot on my bucket list. I am going to
live every day to the fullest and make the
best of it. It is all good and it will get
better...."

1970
I worked at the the Chrysler Eldon
Avenue Gear and Axle plant on July 15th,
1970.

July 15th, 1970 was a very hot day.
I asked for a heat pass three times.

The union contract allowed for a heat
pass when the temperature was above 90^0.

The foreman kept delaying. I understood
that he was waiting for it to cool down so
that he could refuse.

I had family call in a family emergency.

I told family that if they asked what the
emergency was, just say it is personal, as
the union contract did not require

personal information to justify a family emergency.

The foreman came and told me there was a family emergency.

He gave me the look, but he couldn't do anything about it.

When I arrived at home twenty minutes later, the phone was ringing.

When I answered the phone, it was my mother.

I asked,
"why are you calling? I am supposed to be at work."

She answered,
"Didn't you hear? Three people were just shot dead where you work."

I answered,
"no, I don't have a radio in my car."

What happened is as follows.
Mr. James Johnson worked in department, 78, the Brake Shoe Dept.
On July 15, 1970 Mr. James Johnson was

taken off his job as a conveyer loader and replaced by someone with two weeks seniority in violation of the union contract.

Mr. Johnson had seniority and could not be replaced by someone without seniority according to the union contract.

He was switched to a brake oven job, where he worked in 120, degree heat.

Mr. James Johnson went into the labor relations' office with a foreman and a union steward to object to the violation of his rights according to the union contract.

He was suspended on the spot for insubordination and security guards escorted Mr. James Johnson out of the plant.

Mr. James Johnson then returned to the plant with an M1 Carbine loaded with a banana clip and shot and killed two foremen and a job setter.

He was arrested and tried for murder.

The jury voted for acquittal.

Mr. James Johnson was not guilty, "by reason of temporary insanity."

He was sent to a state hospital.

He was released from the state hospital.

After that Mr. James Johnson sued Chrysler Corporation for violation of the union contract resulting in temporary insanity and the three homicides.

On May 12, 1973, James Johnson was awarded workman's compensation for the injuries done to him by Chrysler, $75 a week, retroactive to the day of the killing, July 15th, 1970.

Read the following for more interesting details of that case including details of the jury trial:

Chapter 4 Black Rage 1971: The Case of James Johnson, Jr.pp. 81-111 (31 pages)
https://www.jstor.org/stable/j.ctt9qggtn.8
1971

August 14–20, 1971:
The Stanford prison experiment (SPE) recruited ordinary college students to examine the psychological effects of perceived power in the context of a prison setting with guards and prisoners.

The experiment had to be stopped because the guards became sadistic, and the prisoners became traumatized.

I thought about James Johnson and the harsh work environment at the Chrysler Eldon Avenue Gear and Axle Plant.

Training in Psychiatry 1972-1975

1972
In 1972 I started my first year in training to become a psychiatrist.

I was taught the basic principles of psychotherapy and psychoanalysis.

I learned about transference and countertransference.

In transference the patient projects his life's experience onto the psychiatrist.

In countertransference the psychiatrist projects his life experience onto the patient.

During treatment the patient learns to see the psychiatrist for what the psychiatrist is.

The patient learns to separate his past experiences from his present experiences.

During the process the goal is to learn to function effectively and to discard learning from the past that leads to repetitive errors and depression, anxiety, anger, and other emotions that impair quality of life.

The psychiatrist learns to discard past learning that impairs his ability to see the patient clearly for what the patient is and not to confuse the patient with people the psychiatrist has encountered in the past.

It is difficult to learn to diagnose mental illness because mental illness is complex and abstract.

Every patient at Lafayette Clinic was an experimental subject.

All patients had to sign consent to be participants in medical and psychiatric research before they could be admitted for evaluation and treatment.

Patients were evaluated for four to six weeks before their medications were started.

They were tested in many ways.

One test, the Minnesota Multiphasic Personality Inventory (MMPI), is a psychological test.

The MMPI in 1972 asked if you did or did not avoid touching a door handle.

If you avoided touching a door handle you were given a high score in on the paranoia scale.

The current version is the The MMPI-2, which has 567 true-false questions and takes approximately 60 to 90 minutes to complete.

The current version does not include the question about avoiding door handles.

This is because the culture has changed.

We are now constantly washing hands and very conscious of spreading germs in health care facilities and public places.

Mental illness is shaped by culture.

Patients were also presented at multiple training and research conferences where all of the testing was reviewed, and a diagnosis and treatment strategy was formulated.

One patient was diagnosed as having schizophrenia at one conference.

At a later conference the same patient was diagnosed with Bipolar Disorder.

I attended both conferences and I was confused.

I mentioned the fact that the same patient was previously diagnosed as having schizophrenia. I was confused and I was seeking information to end increase my understanding and end my confusion.

The response was unexpected and hostile
and implied that I was merely a, "troublemaker."

I did not receive the information needed
to resolve my confusion.

My confusion merely increased.

In 1973 Lafayette Clinic was going to
become a pioneer in psychosurgery for
the treatment of violent behavior.

John Boaz was a senior resident in
psychiatry.

He was a genius. He graduated AOA, at
the top of his medical school class.

He had blown off the index and middle
finger of his right hand with a blasting
cap. He told me that was why he went into
psychiatry instead of surgery.

He asked me if I wanted to meet
somebody during lunch hour.
I said sure.
It was a warm spring day, and we walked
from Lafayette Clinic, across the Chrysler
Freeway, to a lawyer's office.

This is where I met Gabe Kaimowitz.

Dr. John Boaz talked about experimental psychosurgery, and he compared it to what happened in the concentration camps in Germany in World War II.

I suspect that the conversation was tape recorded, or that Gabe Kaimowitz had a photographic memory.

If you read the opinion in Kaimowitz v. Department of Mental Health for the State of Michigan, the opinion was in large part a transcript of what John Boaz told Gabe Kaimowitz, minus the F bombs and curses that were plentiful in John Boaz's diatribe before Gabe Kaimowitz.

My contribution to the conversation was occurred when John Boaz was done and Gabe Kaimowitz looked at me and asked, "and what do you think."

I responded,
"I agree in principle, but I don't think that the F-bombs and cursing should be included because it will be used to discredit the substance of John's thoughts."

You should review:
KAIMOWITZ v. DEPARTMENT OF
MENTAL HEALTH FOR THE STATE OF
MICHIGAN. No. 73·19434·AW (Mich. Cir.
Ct., Wayne County, July 10, 1973).

This case had a huge impact on
psychiatry and stopped experimental
research in state hospitals and prisons as
it was decided that prisoners and court
committed mental patients lacked the
legal capacity to consent to participation
in medical experiments.

Psychosurgery for control of violent
behavior was dead in its tracks.

Psychosurgery joined the lobotomy as
outside the scope of mainstream
medicine.

1975
I was at the Hawthorn center in 1974 -
1975 doing a rotation in child psychiatry.
Dr. Ralph D. Rabinovitch and his wife, Dr.
Sara Dubo, founded the the Hawthorn
Center in 1956.

The Hawthorn Center was a State
Hospital in Michigan, and the first in the

country to have a comprehensive program that included outpatient, inpatient, day school, research and training programs for disturbed children.

Dr. Ralph Rabinovitch became very prominent as an innovator in child psychiatry.

He presented an unpublished study for the treatment of self-mutilation, such as displayed in Lesch-Nyhan patients.

He did not say where or when the study was conducted. He did not identify the patients.

In that study, cattle prods were used to discourage self-injury in children manifesting self-mutilation.

The unexpected result was that the children would grab the cattle prods and would not let go.

Apparently, it hurt so good that they wanted more.

Needless to say, the experiment was stopped.

Needless to say, cattle prods for children joined lobotomies and psychosurgery as outside the scope of mainstream medication.

At that time my thoughts were that the pain and pleasure centers of the brain were not connected correctly in these patients.

My thought was that the pleasure center was attached to the pain center and injuries must feel good.

While writing this article my thoughts on Lesch-Nyhan have changed.

I am now thinking that in Lesch-Nyhan Disease pain is attached to the powerful reward of sexual gratification.

I am thinking that Lesch-Nyhan patients experience pain as a sexual orgasm, making it impossible to treat.

My thought is that it will be necessary to do psychosurgery and destroy the sexual orgasm center of the brain to stop patients with Lesch-Nyhan Disease from self-mutilating.

I learned about Munchhausen Disorder.

The Munchhausen patient persistently, and intentionally acts as if he or she has a physical or mental illness when he or she does not have a physical or mental illness.

Munchhausen patients may intentionally mutilate themselves to present as mentally or physically ill.

In Munchhausen by proxy, parents persistently, and intentionally act as if their child have a physical or mental illness when the child does not have a physical or mental illness.

The parents may mutilate the child and then bring the child to a doctor to prove that the child has a physical or mental illness.

Munchhausen by Proxy is not uncommon.

Munchausen Disorder is difficult to treat as the patients do not view themselves as mentally ill and refuse treatment when offered.

It is sometimes necessary to place children into foster care to protect them from Munchhausen by Proxy.

They need protection from doctors.

"Protect the patient from doctors?" Did I really write that?

1975
In 1975 I read about the Borderline Personality Disorder.

Borderline patients were identified by finding treatment failures for many mental illnesses.
Among the treatment failures, the author eliminated all the patients that had a known diagnosis.

The treatment failures without a known diagnosis were examined and given the label of Borderline Personality Disorder based upon common symptoms.

Among the symptoms of the Borderline Personality Disorder was a pattern of self-cutting.

Sometimes the pattern was called, "delicate-cutting."

The unfortunate part of the, "delicate cutting," was that about 15% of the patients eventually were successful in committing suicide.

The 15% successful suicide rate was the same 15% successful suicide rate that I had read about in drug addiction, alcoholism and depression. That was in the 1970's.

The common 15% death rate raises the possibility that borderline personality, drug addiction and alcoholism are all part of the same disease.

There is in fact a great deal of overlap among these diseases. They are commonly diagnosed as concurrent or co-existing diseases.

Until we can map these diseases on the 100 billion neurons and a trillion synapses we are only speculating as to the nature and extent of the relationships among borderline personality disorder, drug addiction and depression.

I read a neurology textbook in preparation for the written and oral examinations by the American Board of Psychiatry and Neurology.

The neurology book described a man who had a head injury. After the head injury he did not believe that his arm was his arm.

He cut the arm off. The pain was not his pain.

This was a case of anosognosia.

The failure to recognize a part of your body as your own, your memories as your own, your thoughts as your own, your imagination as your own is called anosognosia.

There are many parts of the brain involved in self-awareness that when damaged can cause anosognosia.

Damage to the following parts of the brain have been implicated in anosognosia: the superior temporal and inferior parictal cortex, basal ganglia, thalamus, putamen, anterior limb of the internal capsule, medial or lateral part of the pons (medial or lateral pontine reticular nuclei), right thalamus, fronto-parietal lesions, basal ganglia or insula, dorsal premotor cortex (BA6), BA44, somatosensory area, primary motor cortex, BA46, insula, inferior parietal lobule, and the right posterior insula.

I was treating a patient who had been brought into my office by his mother.

He was about eight years old.

After about three weeks the treatment was going nowhere.

The mother reported that the patient was suffering from mental illness.

She explained that there was a divorce and the child was suffering a great deal of stress.

After a few weeks I could not identify any symptoms in the child.

I asked,
"why are you coming in for treatment?"

The child answered,
"my parents are getting a divorce and my mom is mad at my dad."

I looked at his mother for her thoughts.

She became very angry and left my office, taking the child with her.

She never returned.

This was an example of Munchhausen by Proxy.

The mother wanted the child to be diagnosed with a mental illness caused by stress from an unfit father.

When I could not find mental illness, she left with the child.
I completed training in Psychiatry in 1975 and started my career as a psychiatrist in Detroit, Michigan.

The Practice of Psychiatry
1975 to the Present
1977
I worked at Henry Ford Hospital from 1975 to 1977.

Dr. Bresnahan, Dr. Pope and I did every third consultation with the medical surgical services from 1975 to 1976.

There were over 800 consultations with the medical surgical services each year.

Dr. Bresnahan resigned in 1976 and in 1976 to 1977 Dr. Pope and I did every other psychiatric consultation.

From 1975 to 1977 I did about 686 consultations with the medical surgical services at Henry Ford Hospital.

I had a quite few terminally ill cancer patients and we dealt with Dr. Elisabeth Kübler-Ross's five stages of death and dying on many levels.

For the pain I often prescribed Brompton's mixture.
My recipe for Brompton's mixture included the usual morphine and cocaine; to which I added Thorazine at night for anxiety, insomnia, and hallucinations; Elavil at night for depression; and methamphetamine in the morning so that the patients could be alert and say their good bye's to their friends and relatives.

With this recipe for Brompton's mixture, and my counseling, my patients did not display any self-mutilation during their grief process.

I needed two years of clinical experience before I could take my oral and written examinations to be board certified in the practice of psychiatry and neurology.

1977
With two years of clinical experience in 1977, I was allowed to take written and oral tests, monitored by the American Board of psychiatry and neurology.

The oral examination addressed the issue of the borderline personality disorder which was a new topic and not in the textbooks.

I suppose that topic was chosen to see if the candidates for certification in psychiatry and neurology were keeping up with the current literature.

I had read about Borderline Personality and passed the oral and written examination.

The most interesting thing about
Borderline Personality Disorder was how
it was originally identified.

The author looked at a collection of
treatment failures.

He looked at patients that had failed to
respond to all kinds of medications and
psychotherapies.

He then eliminated all the patients with a
specific diagnosis.

The patients that were treatment failures
without a known diagnosis were then
given the diagnosis of Borderline
Personality Disorder.

These patients continue to fail to respond
to all kinds of medications and
psychotherapies.

Borderline Personality Disorders are
frequent visitors to hospital emergency
rooms and psychiatric hospitals.
Borderline Personality Disorder patients
are frequent callers to Suicide
Intervention Hotlines and Crisis
Intervention Hotlines.

I recited what I had read about Borderline Personality Disorders and I was certified by the American Board of Psychiatry and Neurology to practice Psychiatry and Neurology in April of 1977.

Since 1977 suicide, homicide and grave disability have become the basis for admission to a psychiatric hospital.

If the patient is not suicidal, not homicidal or not gravely disabled the patient can safely be treated outside of a psychiatric hospital.

The insurance company will not pre-authorize the admission and will not pay for the admission and treatment of that patient if the patient can safely be treated outside of a psychiatric hospital.

If you are admitted to a psychiatric hospital the psychiatrist gives you a diagnosis of mental illness and describes the mental illness as suicidal, homicidal or gravely disabled to qualify for payment by the insurance policy.

Self-mutilation is a basis for suicidal and grave disability.

Therefore, self-mutilation allows for admission and treatment in the hospital and payment by the medical insurance companies.

Grave disability is severe impairment in the ability to take care of oneself.

The patient who is gravely disabled cannot safely receive psychiatric treatment outside of a psychiatric hospital.

If you are a patient in a psychiatric hospital your roommate is suicidal, homicidal or gravely disabled and not safely treated outside of a psychiatric hospital.

Every day, patients and staff are assaulted by patients in psychiatric hospitals. I have been assaulted many times.

1978
Ted Bundy broke into the Chi Omega sorority house at Florida State University,

attacked four, killing two on January 14, 1978.

1984
I went to the Southwestern Indiana Mental Health Center in Evansville, Indiana to be the Medical Director.

At that time, I did not find the treatments of mental illness as very effective.

My clients on average did not find the treatment very effective.

About half of my patients were not taking their medications for a variety of reasons.

Cost, side effects and lack of benefits were the primary reasons.

I had one patient who was suicidal and waited in Welborn Hospital for eight months or more for a transfer to the Evansville State Psychiatric Hospital.

The transfer was supposed to happen in thirty days, but the state hospital balked.

The patient was transferred after eight months, and about a month after he transferred, he was given a weekend pass to spend with his parents.

He hung himself in his bedroom during that weekend pass.

It was put into the newspapers and the staff told me about it.

He was what we call an outlier.

Most suicidal episodes resolve within the first week or two.

His suicidal episode had not resolved in almost a year. That unusually long period of suicidal risk made him an outlier.

He was outside the usual time period for a suicidal episode to resolve.

There is no blood test or x-ray or objective test to determine when a suicidal episode has resolved.

It is a judgment call on the part of the psychiatrist, as to when it is safe to release a suicidal patient from continuous observation to independent living.

I had another patient who was homicidal.

He was brought into the hospital by the police because of homicidal behavior.

He remained homicidal for six weeks so that I had him in bed restraints for six weeks.

He was also an outlier.

Patients usually resolve their homicidal tendencies within less than twenty-four hours.

He, however, was in restraints for six weeks and threatened homicide daily for six weeks.

One day he changed abruptly, like somebody had turned off the switch. He apologized for threatening to kill me daily for six weeks.

He was polite and calm and no longer in a rage.

I forgot what medications I was treating him with.

I don't believe the medications resolved his homicidal episode.

I believe that his illness ran its course.

After a few days, I determined he was safe and stable, and I discharged him.

I was lucky. He did not return and kill me.

I never heard from him again.

He was also an outlier, and only clinical judgment was available to determine when it was safe to release him back ito the community.

1987
In 1987 I entered the world of prison psychiatry.

Prison psychiatry is a very stressful environment.

When I walked onto the unit the Sargeant would announce, "Dr. Yee alert." Apparently, my presence sparked a change in the culture and a change in the behavior of the Correctional Officers.

The change apparently did not last when I left, and returned with another, "Dr. Yee alert."

The Sargeant was very pleasant and polite to me.

But he was not shy about announcing, "Dr. Yee alert."

I never mentioned it to him because I did not want to spark an adversarial relationship.

I was content to work with the Sargeant and the Correctional officers on a friendly basis and encourage small, cumulative changes over time.

In 1987 psychiatrists performed physical examinations as part of the psychiatric admission assessment.

I examined a patient who was transferred from another facility with a diagnosis of, "psychosis."

It was my practice to examine patients physically and mentally immediately upon admission.

We were allowed a window of twenty-four hours to complete the examination and paperwork.

I have developed the practice of error trapping as a part of a risk management strategy in my practice of medicine and psychiatry.

In that sense, I have harnessed my obsessive-compulsive tendencies as an asset.

I had prior experiences where patients were admitted with undiagnosed fractured jaws, undiagnosed fractured legs, undiagnosed tubal pregnancies and undiagnosed acute appendicitis.

If you didn't diagnose the fractures and medical condition immediately upon admission, then legally you owned them as they could have happened after admission.

In each case, I had been lucky, and had diagnosed them immediately, at the time of admission, and had secured an immediate medical intervention with a good result.

That evening, when I examined the patient with the putative diagnosis of, "psychosis," I found the patient to be delirious, with a pneumothorax.

I ordered an immediate medical intervention that resulted in a hospital admission and treatment of a fractured trachea with pneumothorax.

The patient recovered physically.

I lost track of the patient and do not know what happened after that.

Joan Tucker was a nurse, and my supervisor at the time.

Since 1977 my supervisors have been nurses and social workers and psychiatric technicians. Imagine that. I was being managed?

She raised quite a ruckus.
She did not want the prison psychiatric hospital to become the dumping ground for the state's prison system.
This case and the, "Dr. Yee," alerts made me think about The Stanford Prison Experiment (SPE).

Power Corrupts and Absolute Power Corrupts Absolutely is old wisdom, and Biblical in nature.

In 1987. in the Michigan prisons, I had heard reference to, "thump therapy."

The power of the Correctional Officers had made sadistic behaviors such as, "thump therapy," part of the prison culture.

The prisoners responded with a campaign of reprisals against the Correctional Officers.

The prisoners would work in teams to trap Correctional Officers and force the Correctional Officers to give the prisoners sex and drugs.

The prisoners were so successful in this campaign that the Michigan Department of Corrections offered training to new employees that included, "The Anatomy of a Setup."

This training described how prisoners worked in teams to trap Correctional Officers.

Correctional Officers that were caught in these traps did the training and described how prisoners had been successful.

Prisoners were able to force Correctional Officers, Social Workers, Nurses, Doctors and other employees into having sex with prisoners and into smuggling drugs and other things into the prisons for the prisoners.

Sometimes the prison employees reported the situation to their supervisors and were put on probation.

Sometimes the prison employees hid the problem, were caught, prosecuted, and sent to prison.

Sometime between 1987 and 1991 a very violent prisoner was escorted out of his cell.

He had a four-man escort.
As the four correctional officers walked down the corridors of the prison, they passed a porter.

A porter is a prisoner who is allowed out of his cell during the day to work.

The porter might be paid fifty cents an hour. I am not recalling exactly how much they were paid. The money was trivial.

They were outside their cell and they had something to do. Money was hard to get in prison.

At that time the prison had buckets with wire handles.

The porter had removed the wire handle and straightened it out so that it could be used as a weapon or "shank."

Making weapons is an artform among prisoners. Homemade weapons in prison are called shanks.

The porter passed the shank to the violent prisoner with the four-man escort.

The prisoner stabbed one of the Correctional Officers, (CO's), in the four-man escort through the heart with the wire.

This all happened in a second or two. The four-man escort had no time to react until after the stabbing.

The CO who was stabbed assisted in restraining the prisoner and taking the shank from him.

The stabbed CO then passed out and died.

What happened was that after being stabbed through the heart the CO bled into the pericardium.

The pericardium is a fibrous sac with a slippery lining that encloses the heart and allows it to swell and shrink without friction on the surface of the heart.

The Correctional Officer's heart had been punctured and bled into the pericardium.

As the pericardium filled with blood it constricted the heart so that it could not expand and fill up with blood.

Without blood to pump, the heart was not able to maintain blood flow and blood pressure and the CO collapsed and died.

This happened before CO's wore vests. Now CO's wear vests to prevent death by stabbing through the heart or lungs.

Working in prisons is not a simple or easy proposition.

Nothing in medical school prepared me for working in prison.

Living in a trailer park, living in Detroit, and working in Detroit factories prepared me for working in prison.

I reviewed the medical and psychiatric records of many prisoners.

Their records stretched back to childhood.

Their records included treatments in pediatric psychiatric hospitals, adolescent psychiatric hospitals, adult psychiatric hospitals, and substance abuse treatment facilities.

The same patients at various times were diagnosed with schizophrenia, bipolar disorder, schizoaffective disorder borderline personality disorder, antisocial personality disorder and substance abuse and addiction.
I could only conclude that none of the diagnosis were based upon science.

Rather, they were merely based on collections of symptoms that changed over time.

The symptoms were fundamental, and the diagnosis were conjectural.

The symptoms of mental illness are legion.

Symptoms of mental illness include thoughts, behaviors, and emotions.

Specific thought symptoms include hallucinations, paranoia, delusions, obsessions, amnesias, dementias, disorganized thoughts, racing thoughts, poverty of thought, slowed thoughts, anosognosias (the lack of the thought that your arm is your arm or the image in your head is a memory or your imagination), the belief that you have a symptom when you don't have a symptom and the thought that others should think you have a symptom when you don't have a symptom and confusion of thoughts.

Specific emotional symptoms include depression, anxiety, panic, lack of emotion, inappropriate emotions, anger, rage, lack of pleasure (anhedonia), mood swings from high energy to low energy emotional states.

Specific behavioral symptoms include assault, suicide, self-mutilation, compulsive behaviors such as repetitive hand washing, perseveration or continuing on a previous task after a new task is introduced, excessive and binge eating, anorexia or not eating enough, insomnia or not sleeping enough, hypersomnia sleeping too much, avoiding crowds, pulling out hair.

Most "seasoned," or experienced psychiatrists treat symptoms and enter diagnosis into the record to secure insurance payments or because it was required by the employer.

Medicine is one thing, business is another.

I had a patient who went into a homicidal rage in prison.

In prison they call this "Stir Crazy." Island fever, cabin fever, running amok, are descriptions of similar situations.

I put a patient into restrains for six weeks.

When he came out of his rage, I said to him,

"I don't know why you went into the rage. I don't think that my medications had much effect."

"To me, it seemed that your rage ran its course. You came out if it and the medications were not effective."

I asked,

"can you tell me why you went into the rage and how you came hot of it?"

The patient answered,

"I don't know, doc. Every now and then I go on a nut. I can't help it."

"There is nothing I can do. I just stay that way for a while. Then it just goes away."

There were a group of prisoners who would swallow objects.

They knew if they swallowed an object, they would go to a hospital outside of the prison to have it extracted.

A psychiatrist decided to order a laxative instead of sending the patient to the hospital for an extraction.

The plastic spoon formed a bowel obstruction, the laxative caused the spoon to perforate the bowel, and the patient died of an acute peritonitis from the perforated bowels.

After that, patients were always sent to the outside hospital for extraction of foreign objects.

1989
Ted Bundy was executed in Florida in an electric chair.

I thought about, "running amok," my prison work and the patients I placed into restraints during periods of murderous rages.

Ted Bundy displayed episodes of murderous rages.

The criminal justice system did not medicate him, it utilized capital punishment and the electric chair.

The antisocial personality is not a mental illness in the criminal justice system.

1994
Jeffrey Lionel Dahmer, died November 28, 1994. He was murdered by other prisoners.

Pedophiles are considered fair targets in prison. It is the prison culture.

1995
Around 1995 I accepted the position of Medical Director of a nursing home in Warsaw, Indiana.

This nursing home kept its beds filled by accepting any patient offered by another nursing home.
As a result, I found myself providing medical and psychiatric care for about thirty of the most difficult patients I have ever encountered in my practice of medicine.

They included patients with severe brain damage, severely mentally retarded patients with medical and behavioral problems, and two patients with Lesch-Nyhan disease.

I had read about patients with Lesch-Nyhan disease.

It was another thing to look into the empty eye sockets of a patient who had pulled both eyeballs out and had his hands restrained to his waist to prevent continual digging into the empty eye sockets.

I read the medical record. The patient had been offered every medication and treatment without benefit.

He still needed to have his hands restrained to prevent digging into the empty eye sockets.

I had a severely mentally retarded patient.

He would ask for a Coca Cola frequently during the day.When he was told, "no," you and only have two a day."

he would respond by saying, "no," and slapping himself in the face.

In my mind I could see his caretakers saying, "no," and slapping his face.

That is how some mentally retarded patients learn. They mimic what they see and experience.

In his case his caretakers said, "no," and slapped him on the face.

When I said, "no," to him he echoed the, "no," and added the slap to complete his lesson.

There are many reasons why the mentally retarded self-mutilate.

In 2003 I read about Aron Ralston, a man trapped in the mountains, who had to make a choice.

His arm was wedged between two rocks.
For 129 hours he waited for a rescue.
The rescue did not arrive.
Aron Ralston realized he had the choice of dying or cutting his arm off to escape.

Aron Ralston cut his own arm off to from his trap and to escape death.

I don't think that I could cut my own arm off.

That event was made into a movie.

Sometimes self-mutilation makes perfect sense.

Sometimes it doesn't.

2005
Nobel Panel Urged to Rescind Prize for Lobotomies
August 10, 2005 12:00 AM ET
Heard on Day to Day
ERIC WEINER

The lobotomy is now considered barbaric.

This is in large part is due to the excessive use of the procedure because it was so simple and easily used compared to alternative treatment prior to the arrival of Thorazine.

The lesson from all of this is that no

matter how sophisticated and cutting edge your work is now, in the future it will be considered crude and rudimentary.

Proceed with caution and moderation.

Moderation in all things remains good advice.

Zeal and excess are applauded in the moment and vilified in the future.

It is a matter of public record, Coalinga State Hospital opened in August 2005, the first state hospital built in California in 50 years. It cost $388 million dollars to build. It is estimated that it costs $200,000 a year to house a patient in a California State Hospital.

The exact figure is hard to come by.

It is hard to decipher the official accounts of the California State Hospital system. Seventy three percent of Coaling State Hospital patients are violent sexual predators.

I have heard that some of them are treated with Depo-Provera hormone shots to reduce the intensity of their sexual drives.

I have my doubts about any treatment being effective to stop sexual predation.

Sexually violent predators are likely to stay at Coaling State Hospital for a long time.

I have my doubts about depo-provera shots because I have had more than one Klinefelter patient that was a sexual predator.

Klinefelter patients have an extra X chromosome and have high levels of estrogen resulting in males with breasts and large hips.

If this condition does not stop sexual predation, it is not likely that depo provera shots will stop sexual predation.

In general, sexually driven behaviors are not very responsive to treatment. I submit Ted Bundy and Jeffrey Dahmer as poster boys for my premise that sexually driven behaviors are not responsive to psychiatric treatment.

See: "Criminality in men with Klinefelter's Syndrome and XYY syndrome: a Cohort Study," Kirstine Stochholm, Anders Bojesen, Anne Skakkebæk Jensen, Svend Juul, Claus Højbjerg Gravholt

2008
I quit my job and started back into private practice as a contract psychiatrist.

I would be a self-employed contractor.

Different recruiters would, "find," contracts and take part of my hourly wage for finding the contract.

I was in fact paying for the right to work without benefits. Imagine that.
I had read about Kelly Girl Service, Inc. and advertising for temporary office help.
I could not afford their rates.

I didn't realize that the secretaries were paying for their jobs.

Temporary help can be a high paying job, but the recruiter takes a "big slice," of the pie.

Ricky, "Crusher," Cortez died May 16, 2008: at the age of 77 from a sudden heart attack in Garden City, Mich.

In 2008 I was working at Muskegon Prions and Brooks Prison in Muskegon, Michigan. I had a social worker as a supervisor.

While working at these prisons I was assaulted and had a laceration on the occipital, or back part of my scalp. It bled profusely.

There was a lot of blood on my hands and the wall and door of the, "crime scene," It was marked by tape, just like in the movies.

I was told to go to the emergency room.

The emergency room physician said, "I can put three or four stitches in there if you want."

I asked,
"will there be pain?"

He answered,
"Yes, there will be pain."

I asked,
"What will happen if you don't put the stitches in?"

He answered,
"The scar will be larger."

I said,
"I don't like pain. I prefer the larger scar. I don't want any stitches."

"Thank you anyway."

Because I was a contractor without health insurance, I had to pay for the emergency room visit with my own money.

I decided that the next time, I would not go to the emergency room.

When I returned to work the next day, a prisoner told me he had heard about the assault.

He asked if I had been injured.

I was careful not to identify, or say anything about the prisoner who assaulted me.

This could have been part of a set up to get me to violate confidentiality and create an opportunity to blackmail me.

What I said was that my sister hit harder than I was hit in the assault.

I was essentially stating that the prisoner that hit me hit like a girl.

This was a serious insult in the prison community.

The fact that I returned to work the next day without serious injury undermined any credibility for future threats by this prisoner.

Reputation and "respect," is very important in the prison culture among inmates.

I met patients after 2008 who had cut their abdomen open so many times the surgeons were not able to sew it together so that it would heal tightly.

One day I asked one why he had gone to the hospital over the weekend.

He smiled and said, "I was just doing pushups."

That's all it took for his bowels to fall out of his abdomen unto the floor.

He no longer needed to cut himself to create a medical emergency.

Was this Munchhausen's syndrome?

Was this Repetitive Self-Mutilation Syndrome, (RSM)?

Was this Borderline Personality Disorder?

Are these separate mental illnesses or simply many faces of the same mental illness?

We really don't know what mental illness is at the basic level of neurons and synapses of the brain.
We still guess and speculate.

Self-mutilation occurs in many cultures as part of an acceptable display of grief.

Women of the Dani tribe in Papua, New Guinea will cut off the top of their finger to show grief for the loss of a relative, and also, to drive away evil spirits.

Repetitive Self-Mutilation Syndrome, (RSM), is common among students.

Repetitive Self-Mutilation Syndrome, (RSM), is often labeled as parasuicidal behavior.

Self-mutilation can manifest with cutting, scratching, burning, head banging, preventing wounds from healing, picking, poking, and hair pulling.

It can become contagious in schools and will manifest tattooing, and scarification.

Scarification manifests with scratching, etching, burning, and branding. Scarification merges with implants. Tattoos, scarification, and implants are regarded by some as art forms.

However, tattooing, scarification and implants can be viewed through the lens of sadomasochistic behaviors.

Sadomasochism involves pleasure from inflicting or receiving physical or mental suffering from another person.

Sadomasochism can manifest with cutting, scratching, burning, head banging, preventing wounds from healing, picking, poking, and hair pulling, tattooing, scarification, implants, bondage, discipline, dominance or humiliation.

Arguably an abusive supervisor is engaged in sadomasochistic behavior in the workplace to humiliate employees for sexual gratification.

This is often overlooked and is more pervasive than groping and other sexual behaviors in the workplace.

Arguably, the most extreme example of sadomasochism would be gender change surgery.

The surgeon the sadist, the patient the masochist.

Occasionally the patient finds dissatisfaction with gender change surgery. and asks for reverse gender change surgery.

That is a messy proposition for sure.

1% to 8% of patients who start gender change seek a reversal of sex change procedures including surgery.

Gender Dysphoria is a recognized mental illness.

Patients with Gender Dysphoria will often mutilate their genitals.

Many patients with gender dysphoria suffer from concurrent autism spectrum disorder.

Nothing is simple when you are dealing with neurons connected by a complex web of 100 billion neurons and a trillion or more synapses.

This neuron web is exposed to the tidal influences of hormones with widely distributed effects and the influences of culture, and a variety of daily stresses and traumas.

I have been exposed, second hand, to many of these daily stresses and traumas.

Patients reported them to me.

I had patients who claimed to be vampires.

They would bite their partners and suck blood during sexual intercourse.

They may or may not acquire AIDS this way.

I don't know if they had AIDS.

Patients often tell me things to see if I am shocked.

I have been in the business for fifty years. What I have, read, heard and seen was shocking at first.

Now, I have the opinion that if someone can imagine something, it has been done, it is being done, and it will be done many times again.

The current world population is 7.7 billion. All 7.7 billion people are all doing something.

I have been assaulted by patients a number of times.

I was assaulted by a patient who had stabbed a prior psychiatrist in the eye with a pencil.

That patient had also assaulted another psychiatrist in a state hospital.

He punched me in the eye so hard that it pushed the contact lens into the eye socket above the eyeball.

The emergency room physician could not remove it and sent me to an ophthalmologist.
The ophthalmologist removed it.

The ophthalmologist told me I was lucky.

He said that if it had been a hard contact lens, it could have caused a lot of damage to the eyeball.

I have been lucky. I have not been seriously injured.

Self -mutilation, suicide and homicide are often concurrent in the same patient.

I have examined patients that assaulted psychiatrists so severely that the psychiatrists were permanently disabled or died.

These same patients also had histories of suicidal episodes and suicide attempts.

2000
In the year 2000 Gabe Kaimowitz was a crusader subject to bo the applause and scorn. He was an outlier in the practice of law. He was always pushing the envelope. He never strayed onto the middle path. Read the following regarding his activities.

The combustible crusader, By William
Dean Hinton, Jul 5-11, 2000, Vol. 16, No.
27,
https://www.orlandoweekly.com/orlando/t
he-combustible-
crusader/Content?oid=2262584

2003
The Human Genome Project (HGP) was
launched in 1990 and was declared
complete on April 14, 2003.

What I learned from the human genome
project is that the difference in DNA
between any two individuals is 0.6%.

That means when I am looking at a
patient, I am looking at 99.4 percent
myself and 0.6% someone else.

That 99.4 percent is why we are able to
speak the same language and understand
each other.
When we communicate, the 0.6%
difference between us is shared and
modified.
That is the point of psychotherapy,
transference, and countertransference.

The point is for the psychiatrist to gain a greater understanding of mental health, mental illness and the treatment of mental illness.

The point is for the patient to gain a greater understanding of mental health and mental illness.

The goal is to teach the patient how to resolve mental illness and acquire a better handle on mental health and the ability to function effectively in the community.

2012
Dr. John Boaz died 12-11-2012
I tried to find Dr. Boaz. I was sorry to find out that he died before I could contact him.

I found out that the trajectory of Dr. Boaz's life was as complicated as the life of Gabe Kaimowitz.

They were both quite interesting and provoked major changes in psychiatry.
2012

I started working in California State Prisons including Pelican Bay Prison when it was a level 5 Super Max or maximum security prison, CSP-Sac in Folsom, California and San Quentin Prison in San Quentin, California.

I heard a lot of stories while working in these prisons.

California Prisons has many celebrities. I never met any of them.

There were the Menendez brothers who claimed they murdered their parents because they were abused.

There was Charles Manson.

Correctional Officers, (CO's), told me that Charles Manson had the ability to, "get into your head," so that the CO's had to be rotated out of his influence at regular intervals. True? Urban Myth? I don't know.

I saw a gardener quietly working at a prison.

I was told he killed another prisoner with a single punch.

I was told of a cell fight. One prisoner was heard saying, "you hit like a girl," during the fight.

The prisoner who said, "you hit like a girl," was found with his head caved in.

The other prisoner felt compelled to cave in the skull to make sure everyone knew that he did not, "hit like a girl."

Reputation and, "respect," is that important in prison.

"Context," is important.
Prisons have a lot of, "context."

2016
The following was posted on the internet about Gabe Kaimowitz:
The Florida Bar
Member Profile
Gabe Kaimowitz
Last Known Contact Information
PO Box 140119

Gainesville, FL 32614-0119
Office: 352-375-2670
Fax: 352-375-2670
10-Year Discipline History:
Discipline cases that are public record are posted below. Select the reference number to view the Supreme Court Order and other related documents. Members of the public may obtain information about any disciplinary history older than 10 years by emailing LRInfo@floridabar.org or by calling (850) 561-5839. The Media should call the Public Information Department at (850) 561-5666.

Action Date   Reference
Suspended - with Conditions
             11/21/2014   201300238
Disbarment   12/01/2016 201700116
https://www.floridabar.org/directories/find-mbr/profile/?num=633836

I would like to talk to Mr. Gabe Kaimowitz to find out what he recalled about our meeting with John Boaz in 1973.

Gabe Kaimowitz and John Boaz shared genius and lives worthy of a Shakespearean Tragedy.

In December of 2016 I was assaulted while working at Atascadero State Hospital in Atascadero, California.

During 2016 I was told that I was the fourth psychiatrist to be assaulted at Atascadero State Hospital.

The three psychiatrists before me had gone to the emergency room for treatment of injuries.

One psychiatrist had been assaulted ten or more times and was assigned to a job outside of the hospital where he would no longer be exposed to assaults.

I was again told to go to the emergency room by my supervisor.

This time I refused, as I had not received what I considered any serious injury that an emergency room physician could treat.

My blood pressure was elevated at work for a few weeks from traumatic stress.

I worked through the experience without any PTSD, as the experience was not as traumatic as being beaten by my father as a child.

What does not kill you makes you stronger.

I suppose that the patient that assaulted this little old Chinaman suffered a substantial loss of status by the fact that I did not go to the emergency room, I did not miss time from work, and I did not suffer any injuries like the three psychiatrists before me.

2017
I returned to work in a Michigan prison. I was told that a prisoner managed to hold a female CO hostage in a room.

An armored tactical unit came to rescue the CO while she was being raped.

The prisoner told the tactical unit,

"I will kill the bitch if you try to stop me. If you let me finish, I will let her out without hurting her."

This conversation was broadcast throughout the prison on the walkie talkies used by the CO's.

The prisoner raped the woman, and she was released.

The female was married to another CO who heard the conversation as his wife was being raped.

They wound up getting a divorce.

The rule was changed to, "rescue, no discretion, no delay."

I returned to I-Max and entered the personnel office, which was outside the razor wire.

I asked why it was locked because it was not inside the prison walls.

I was told that a prisoner was sent to the emergency room with a boot print on his face.

Three CO's were fired because there was evidence that they had assaulted that prisoner.

There was fear of retaliation.

There is now routine, "Active Shooter," training in prisons and health care facilities.

The reason is that disgruntled employees and patients can return with guns.

There continues to be an undeclared war between prisoners and correctional officers.

Sometimes the hostility occurs between management and line staff in the prison system. Working in prisons is not easy.

Having reviewed my life's experience with self-mutilation, let us consider diagnosis and treatment.

Diagnosis and treatment, nothing is easy.

Mental Illness or Not Mental Illness?

Patients and their families often ask if the patient has a mental illness.

A Little Context Before the Answer

This is a very difficult question to answer on many levels.

Worldwide about one in seven prisoners are psychotic or suffering from clinical depression.

See:
The mental health of prisoners: a review of prevalence, adverse outcomes and interventions
Prof Seena Fazel, MD, Dr Adrian J Hayes, PhD, Katrina Bartellas, BCom, Dr Massimo Clerici, MD, and Prof Robert Trestman, MD
Lancet Psychiatry. Author manuscript; available in PMC 2016 Sep 1.
Published in final edited form as:
Lancet Psychiatry. 2016 Sep; 3(9): 871–881.

Published online 2016 Jul 14. doi:
10.1016/S2215-0366(16)30142-0
PMCID: PMC5008459
EMSID: EMS69411
PMID: 27426440

Medications and treatments did not close prisons.

In fact, California, determined that the treatment of sexually violent predators had been a gross failure.

California expended a great deal of time and money changing the criminal justice system and constructing a state hospital for sexual predators.

In August of 2005, after spending three hundred and eight million dollars, California opened Coalinga State Hospital.

Coalinga State Hospital houses nine hundred and forty one Sexually Violent Predators at a cost of three hundred and eight million dollars for the hospital, plus an estimated $200,000 per year per prisoner for psychiatric treatment, security and other housing maintenance, legal and administrative expenses.

The number of mentally ill in prisons and jails probably exceeds the number of mentally ill that were previously in state hospitals.

About one third of the homeless population is mentally ill.

Having created context, let's examine details.

First, the DSM-V is copyrighted. As copyrighted material, you need to pay the American Psychiatric Association for the right to use it.

As copyrighted material it does not evolve under the scientific method. There is the opportunity for a lot of politics and other influences to shape the DSM-V that is not open to public scrutiny.

For example, at one time homosexuality was considered a mental illness in the DSM-III.

Homosexuality is no longer considered to be a mental illness.

This change was not a change in science, rather it was a change in culture and law.

There used to be paranoid schizophrenia and undifferentiated schizophrenia and disorganized schizophrenia, etc in the DSM-III.

In the DSM-V there is just schizophrenia.

The reason for the change is that over time it was determined that the same patients were diagnosed with paranoid schizophrenia and undifferentiated schizophrenia and disorganized schizophrenia, etc.

It could only be concluded that schizophrenia, for a variety of reasons could appear differently at different times.

I recalled all he charts that I had reviewed that had included schizophrenia, bipolar disorder, schizoaffective disorder, borderline personality disorder and drug abuse and addiction as past diagnosis.

I recalled all the patients who had been examined by two clinicians on the same day and given different diagnosis by the two clinicians.

I recalled being called a troublemaker at Lafayette Clinic for asking why one professor had diagnosed a patient as having schizophrenia and another professor had diagnosed the same patient with Bipolar Disorder.

I can only conclude that current mental illnesses are defined by speculation about collections of symptoms.

The structural and functional abnormalities of the brain that cause symptoms of mental illness have not been identified sufficiently to understand how medications work; or what mental illnesses actually are; or how to cure mental illness.

The brain has 100 billion neurons with more than a trillion synapses.

The neurons and synapses are arranged into a complex web that is not mapped or adequately understood.

We do not understand mental illness, the treatment of mental illness or the cure for mental illness. We still speculate.

Another level to the confusion in diagnosis is the influence of the five stages of grief discussed above.

When the patient has a relapse, the patient enters a grief reaction that includes denial, anger, depression, negotiation, and acceptance.

These stages of the grief reaction to the relapse can occur in any order and any combination. They can all occur in the same day or the same hour.

This can go a long way to explaining why the same patient can be examined by two

clinicians on the same day and have two
diagnosis.

About half of my patients were not taking
their medications as prescribed.

There do not appear to be reliable studies
on medication noncompliance. But 50%
appears to be a common finding.

A patient will be noncompliant if the
benefit is not subjectively very good, the
side effects outweigh the subjective value
of the benefit, or if the cost and effort
exceed the perceived value of the benefits.

The patients vote with their feet.

It would seem better treatments are more
important than strategies compelling the
patient to accept a marginal benefit.

Self-mutilation is not a mental illness
when it is a cultural ritual to become
blood brothers, or cultural ritual to
display grief. Self-mutilation is not a
mental illness when it is used as a tool to
gain status or opportunity.

Self-mutilation is not a mental illness
when it is necessary to cut your own arm
off to save your life.

Self-mutilation is not a mental illness
when it is a culturally accepted art form
such as tattooing, or scarification.

Self-mutilation is a symptom of mental
illness when it is due to Lesch-Nyhan
Disorder, compulsive scratching,
Borderline Personality Disorder,
Repetitive Self-Mutilation Syndrome,
(RSM), Sadomasochism, Gender
Dysphoria, Munchuasen Disorder, or
Munchhausen Disorder by Proxy, etc.

The patient or family often asks if the self-
mutilations can be treated.

The answer given by the doctor, mirrors
the answer given by the lawyer.

Anybody can sue anybody for anything.

Anything can be treated by a psychiatrist.

A more complete answer is, you can sue

anybody for anything, but you often incur a lot of expenses and lose the lawsuit.

A more complete answer is, you can treat anything, but sometimes you are worse off after the treatment than before the treatment started.

People can die from allergies to medications and other medication side effects.

Often the side effects of the treatments are worse than the mental illness being treated.

The family that wants a two-year-old treated for gender dysphoria presents a complex medical and psychiatric and ethical dilemma.

Does the two-year old truly have gender dysphoria or do the parents have gender dysphoria regarding the child?

Another way to frame the question, "is this a case of Munchhausen by Proxy?"

The family members will often press to treat the patient when the patient does not want to be treated.

The competent patient can say no.

The patient who has a court appointed legal guardian can say no, but the legal guardian can force the treatment upon the patient.

The psychiatrist can refuse to treat the patient when the patient says no, and the legal guardian says yes.

The psychiatrist can tell the legal guardian to find another psychiatrist to perform the treatment that the patient wants to refuse.

For an introduction and overview of the treatment of violence see:

"Violence, mental illness, and the brain –
A brief history of psychosurgery: Part 1 –
From trephination to lobotomy,"
Miguel A. Faria, Jr.
Surg Neurol Int. 2013; 4: 49.

Published online 2013 Apr 5. doi:
10.4103/2152-7806.110146
PMCID: PMC3640229
PMID: 23646259

What are the Treatments of Self-Mutilation?

The treatments for self-mutilation are the treatments for the medical and psychiatric disorder that cause the self-mutilation.

Munchhausen and Munchhausen by Proxy are very difficult to treat.

My experience is that when you tell the patient or the parents what the diagnosis is, they stop coming and find another psychiatrist.

That has been my experience from 1975 to the present.

I have never been successful in treating Munchhausen and Munchhausen by Proxy.

Munchhausen is classified under
factitious disorders.

There is not much information on the
treatment of factitious disorder. No
specific treatment is known to be effective
for Munchhausen and Munchhausen by
Proxy or factitious disorder in general.
See:
Management of Factitious Disorders: A
Systematic Review, Eastwood S. · Bisson
J.I., Psychother Psychosom 2008;77:209–
218, https://doi.org/10.1159/000126072

Lesh-Nyhan disease is is caused by a
mutation in the HPRT1 gene located on
the X chromosome.

The mother carries the defective gene on
one of her two X chromosome and gives it
to half of her sons.

It is a recessive gene and manifests in
males.
It only manifests with females when both
the mother and the father has the X
chromosome with the Lesch-Nyhan trait.

This is rare, men with Lesch-Nyhan disorder rarely have children.

Lesch–Nyhan disease is caused by a deficiency of the enzyme hypoxanthine-guanine phosphoribosyltransferase (HGPRT).

This deficiency occurs in about 1 in 380,000 live births.[2]

I have not been successful in the treatment of Lesch-Nyhan syndrome.

I have not been able to locate an effective treatment for Lesch-Nyhan disease.
See:
Treatment of motor and behavioural symptoms in three Lesch-Nyhan patients with intrathecal baclofen., Orphanet Pozzi, M., Piccinini, L., Gallo, M. et al. J Rare Dis 9, 208 (2014).
https://doi.org/10.1186/s13023-014-0208-3

I have had limited success in the treatment of the mentally retarded. Naltrexone and clomipramine have been tried and have not been better than placebo in at least one study. See:

Pharmacological interventions for self-injurious behaviour in adults with intellectual disabilities: Abridged republication of a Cochrane systematic review, A Gormez, F Rana, S VargheseFirst Published April 30, 2014, https://doi.org/10.1177/0269881114531665 Risperidone has been reported to be effective with self-injurious behaviors.

See:
Pharmacotherapy of disruptive behavior in mentally retarded subjects: A review of the current literature, Frank Häßler Olaf Reis, Developmental Disabilities Research Reviews, 27 October 2010
https://doi.org/10.1002/ddrr.119

I have treated many mentally retarded with behavior disorders.

I have reviewed their records from childhood through adult life in psychiatric hospitals, outpatient clinics and residential facilities.

The records of the mentally retarded reveal multiple therapeutic trials with multiple mood stabilizers, multiple antipsychotics, multiple antidepressants, multiple psychostimulants, naltrexone, Prazosin, Dilantin and multiple seizure medications.

They have been treated with DBT, CBT, individual and group therapies and all the treatments were failures and the mentally retarded are likely to spend the rest of their lives on many more therapeutic trials.

I have treated many borderline patients.

I have treated borderline patients in outpatient clinics, hospitals, and prisons.

In the nineteen eighties the Michigan Department of Mental Health called for a statewide meeting on how best to address the issue of borderline patients in hospitals, emergency rooms and outpatient clinics.

The reason was that the borderline patients were a small minority of patients utilizing a large percentage of the state resources in the outpatient clinics, hospitals and emergency rooms.

This is 2020 and borderline patients continue to be a minority of patients that use a large percentage of resources in hospitals, emergency rooms and outpatient clinics.

I have viewed their records of treatment since childhood and their records are very similar to the records of the treatments of the mentally retarded patients.

They have had many interventions in outpatient clinics, emergency rooms, and hospitals. They have been given the opportunity to try all the medications in the pharmacy and all the individual and group therapies known including DBT, Dialectical Behavioral Therapy, and CBT, Cognitive Behavioral Therapy.

Borderline Patients and Antisocial Personalities in general tend to grow out of their mental illness rather than respond to treatment interventions.

Borderline and Antisocial Personalities tend to grow out of their mental illness between the ages of thirty and forty in half the patients that I have treated since

1972. See:
Meta Analysis Cochrane Review
"Defining borderline patients: An
overview. The American Journal of
Psychiatry," Gunderson, J. G., & Singer,
M. T. (1975). 132(1), 1–10.
https://doi.org/10.11Tre76/ajp.132.1.1

See also, "Characteristics of Borderline
Personality Disorder in a Community
Sample: Comorbidity, Treatment
Utilization, and General Functioning,"
Rachel L. Tomko, MA; Timothy J. Trull,
PhD; Phillip K. Wood, PhD; Kenneth J.
Sher, PhD
Additional Information
Journal of Personality Disorders: Vol. 28,
No. 5, pp. 734-750.
https://doi.org/10.1521/pedi_2012_26_093

See also, "Comorbidity, Treatment
Utilization, and General Functioning,"
Rachel L. Tomko, MA; Timothy J. Trull,
PhD; Phillip K. Wood, PhD; Kenneth J.
Sher, PhD, Journal of Personality
Disorders: Vol. 28, No. 5, pp. 734-750.
https://doi.org/10.1521/pedi_2012_26_093

Transgender patients tend to have issues with quality of life.

See.
"Quality of life of treatment-seeking transgender adults: A systematic review and meta-analysis," Anna Nobili, Cris Glazebrook, and Jon Arcelus, Rev Endocr Metab Disord. 2018; 19(3): 199–220. Published online 2018 Aug 18. doi: 10.1007/s11154-018-9459-y PMCID: PMC6223813 PMID: 30121881

There is an overlap among patients with Gender Dysphoria and Autism Spectrum Disorder,

See
Gender Dysphoria and Autism Spectrum Disorder: A Systematic Review of the Literature, Glidden D., Bouman W.P., Jones B.A., Arcelus J. (2016) Sexual Medicine Reviews, 4 (1) , pp. 3-14.

At this time, all the medications and psychotherapeutic interventions are being offered for the treatment of Munchhousen, Munchhausen by Proxy and Factitious Disorder

There is no literature with robust evidence for the effectiveness of any treatment of factitious disorder.

See:
Management of Factitious Disorders: A Systematic Review, Eastwood S. · Bisson J.I., Psychother Psychosom 2008;77:209–218, https://doi.org/10.1159/000126072

Seasoned psychiatrists treat hallucinations, paranoia, and delusions with antipsychotic medications.

Seasoned psychiatrists treat anxiety with serotonin reuptake inhibitors (SRI's) such as Zoloft, or with beta blockers such as propranolol, or buspirone.

Seasoned psychiatrists treat depression, with serotonin reuptake inhibitors (SRI's) such as Zoloft, or Wellbutrin or Effexor, or Electro Shock Therapy.
Seasoned psychiatrists treat high energy states with lithium, Depakote, Zyprexa, Thorazine and other mood stabilizers.

Newer treatments include electrodes implanted into the brain, and Ketamine (Spravato), which is given as a nasal spray.

Seasoned psychiatrists treat assault, suicide, self-mutilation, with all of the above treatments as generally high energy is involved and brief psychotic and agitated depressive states drive suicide, assault and self-mutilation.

Putting a patient to sleep tends to accelerate the resolution of acute, high-energy psychotic and depressed states that drive suicide, assault and self-mutilation.

The emergency room often relies on racemic ketamine, which is most often given as an infusion into the bloodstream.

This is sometimes called intravenous, or IV, ketamine. It is easily used and rapidly effective.

This psychiatric consultation must end at some arbitrary point.

Thank you for your time and attention. William Yee M.D., J.D., Board Certified Psychiatrist practicing without interruption since 1972 in Michigan, Indiana, Kentucky and California and recently licensed to practice in Texas, at your service.

"Preexisting text," includes names of people and corporations, names of law cases, and text of statutes cited, the titles of articles and books and the content of articles and books cited in the text the prior seventy-nine pages.

My copyright claim is a clam to the "original text," which is my personal experiences as described in the text above and my commentary on the people and corporations, law cases, and text of statutes cited, the articles and books and the content of articles and books cited in the text above.

Preexisting text in this consultation includes but is not limited to the following:

1.
He was bad, so they put an ice pick in his brain..., Elizabeth Day, The Guardian, The Obser1633-1637 ver Neuroscience, Sun 13 Jan 2008 18.40 EST,
https://www.theguardian.com/science/2008/jan/13/neuroscience.medicalscience
2.
10 Awful Realities Behind The Lobotomy Craze," GREGORY MYERS, HUMANS | NOVEMBER 20, 2014,
https://listverse.com/2014/11/20/10-awful-realities-behind-the-lobotomy-craze/
3.
The Eternal Search; the Story of Man and his Drugs by Richard R. Mathison, 1958
On Death and Dying: What the Dying Have to Teach Doctors, Nurses, Clergy and Their Own Families, Elisabeth Kubler-Ross, 1969
4.
Stanford prison experiment (SPE)
Chapter 4 Black Rage 1971: The Case of James Johnson, Jr.pp. 81-111 (31 pages)
https://www.jstor.org/stable/j.ctt9qggtn.8

5.
The Minnesota Multiphasic Personality Inventory (MMPI)
6.
KAIMOWITZ v. DEPARTMENT OF MENTAL HEALTH FOR. THE STATE OF MICHIGAN. No. 73·19434·AW. (Mich. Cir. Ct., Wayne County, July 10, 1973).
7.
"The Anatomy of a Setup." Criminality in men with Klinefelter's Syndrome and XYY syndrome: a Cohort Study," Kirstine Stochholm, Anders Bojesen, Anne Skakkebæk Jensen, Svend Juul, Claus Højbjerg Gravholt
The combustible crusader, By William Dean Hinton, Jul 5-11, 2000, Vol. 16, No. 27,
https://www.orlandoweekly.com/orlando/the-combustible-crusader/Content?oid=2262584
8.
The Human Genome Project (HGP)
9.
The Florida Bar, Member Profile, Gabe Kaimowitz
10."Violence, mental illness, and the brain – A brief history of psychosurgery: Part 1

– From trephination to lobotomy,"
Miguel A. Faria, Jr.
Surg Neurol Int. 2013; 4: 49.
Published online 2013 Apr 5. doi:
10.4103/2152-7806.110146
PMCID: PMC3640229
PMID: 23646259
11.
Management of Factitious Disorders: A
Systematic Review, Eastwood S. · Bisson
J.I., Psychother Psychosom 2008;77:209–
218, https://doi.org/10.1159/000126072
12.
Treatment of motor and behavioural
symptoms in three Lesch-Nyhan patients
with intrathecal baclofen., Orphanet
Pozzi, M., Piccinini, L., Gallo, M. et al. J
Rare Dis 9, 208 (2014).
https://doi.org/10.1186/s13023-014-0208-3
13.
Pharmacological interventions for self-
injurious behaviour in adults with
intellectual disabilities: Abridged
republication of a Cochrane systematic
review, A Gormez, F Rana, S
VargheseFirst Published April 30, 2014,
https://doi.org/10.1177/0269881114531665
14.
Pharmacotherapy of disruptive behavior

in mentally retarded subjects: A review of the current literature, Frank Häßler Olaf Reis, Developmental Disabilities Research Reviews, 27 October 2010 https://doi.org/10.1002/ddrr.119 Meta Analysis Cochrane Review

"Defining borderline patients: An overview. The American Journal of Psychiatry," Gunderson, J. G., & Singer, M. T. (1975). 132(1), 1–10. https://doi.org/10.11Tre76/ajp.132.1.1

15.
See also, "Characteristics of Borderline Personality Disorder in a Community Sample: Comorbidity, Treatment Utilization, and General Functioning," Rachel L. Tomko, MA; Timothy J. Trull, PhD; Phillip K. Wood, PhD; Kenneth J. Sher, PhD

16.
Additional Information
Journal of Personality Disorders: Vol. 28, No. 5, pp. 734-750. https://doi.org/10.1521/pedi_2012_26_093

17.
See also, "Comorbidity, Treatment Utilization, and General Functioning," Rachel L. Tomko, MA; Timothy J. Trull,

PhD; Phillip K. Wood, PhD; Kenneth J. Sher, PhD, Journal of Personality Disorders: Vol. 28, No. 5, pp. 734-750. https://doi.org/10.1521/pedi_2012_26_093
18.
"Quality of life of treatment-seeking transgender adults: A systematic review and meta-analysis," Anna Nobili, Cris Glazebrook, and Jon Arcelus, Rev Endocr Metab Disord. 2018; 19(3): 199–220. Published online 2018 Aug 18. doi: 10.1007/s11154-018-9459-y PMCID: PMC6223813 PMID: 30121881
19.
Gender Dysphoria and Autism Spectrum Disorder: A Systematic Review of the Literature, Glidden D., Bouman W.P., Jones B.A., Arcelus J. (2016) Sexual Medicine Reviews, 4 (1) , pp. 3-14.
20.
Management of Factitious Disorders: A Systematic Review, Eastwood S. · Bisson J.I., Psychother Psychosom 2008;77:209–218, https://doi.org/10.1159/000126072
21.
The mental health of prisoners: a review of prevalence, adverse outcomes and interventions

Prof Seena Fazel, MD, Dr Adrian J Hayes,
PhD, Katrina Bartellas, BCom, Dr
Massimo Clerici, MD, and Prof Robert
Trestman, MD
Lancet Psychiatry. Author manuscript;
available in PMC 2016 Sep 1.
Published in final edited form as:
Lancet Psychiatry. 2016 Sep; 3(9): 871–881.
Published online 2016 Jul 14. doi:
10.1016/S2215-0366(16)30142-0
PMCID: PMC5008459
EMSID: EMS69411
PMID: 27426440

www.ingramcontent.com/pod-product-compliance
Lightning Source LLC
Chambersburg PA
CBHW022007170526
45157CB00003B/1183